For Life:
Defending the Unborn

eicc
publications

Some of the material in this book is based on content previously published in Jubilee, Winter 2013 by the Ezra Institute for Contemporary Christianity, and on content published electronically at www.ezrainstitute.ca.

Published by EICC Publications, a ministry of the Ezra Institute for Contemporary Christianity, 9 Hewitt Ave., Toronto, ON M6R 1Y4

Contributions by Linda Baartse, Joseph Boot and Scott Masson. Copyright of the authors, 2017. All rights reserved. This book may not be reproduced, in whole or in part, without the written permission of the publishers.

Unless otherwise noted, Scripture quotations are taken from the English Standard Version © 2001 by Crossway Bibles, a division of Good News Publishers. Used by permission.

Edited by Ryan Eras.

For volume discounts please contact the Ezra Institute for Contemporary Christianity: info@ezrainstitute.ca; (416)-466-8819, ext. 309.

For Life: Defending the Unborn
ISBN: 978-0-9947279-8-5

For Life: Defending the Unborn

CONTENTS

Introduction 5

Precious Thoughts and Precious Life
in a Culture of Death 11

The Cosmology of Killing:
Moloch Worship Repackaged 30

The Cosmology of Life and Compassion 48

INTRODUCTION

Typically, those of us concerned with the preservation of innocent life in the womb, reflecting the compassion and concern of our maker, start by approaching the issues with pragmatic considerations. We speak of the negative health consequences of abortion, or reason scientifically by showing that the unborn child is, from conception, a human life, and that killing the child is merely a form of murder. Important and significant as these arguments are (and they must be made), many modern pro-abortion intellectuals increasingly *do not* attempt to deny these charges, and appear unconcerned by them. Camille Paglia, a social commentator and pro-abortion writer, has stated, "I have always frankly admitted that abortion is murder, the extermination of the powerless by the powerful, which results in the annihilation of concrete individuals and not just clumps of insensate tissue."[1]

Paglia sees clearly that her ideology constitutes a new *cosmology*, a new social order, based on the autonomy of choice and the absoluteness of man's will and desire, which is beyond good and evil; it is a denial of transcendent law. Such a perspective of absolute autonomy is informed by essentially *religious* considerations. It is insufficient, then, for us to approach and argue the issues only pragmatically, and be dismissed as mere moralizers. We must begin theologically and philosophically. This is the way in which we can show that abortion is not simply a war of words or wills, but a dispute about the nature of reality itself.

Cosmology refers to *order,* or *structure.* It is the way in which we look at and understand the order of our world. It considers the big picture of reality and the implications which flow from it. When we say, as Christians, that abortion is murder, we are not only making an ethical statement, we are also making a statement about some of the most foundational questions about life, such as What is a human being? What is God? and How ought we to live in this world?

When we say that our opposition to abortion is based on our Christian beliefs, we are making a statement about the nature of God and His Word. In that Word, Jesus tells us that murder is a heart issue: "from within, out of the heart of man, come evil thoughts, sexual immorality, theft, murder, adultery, coveting, wickedness, deceit, sensuality, envy, slander, pride, foolishness. All these evil things come from within, and they defile a person" (Mark 7:21-23).

Consider this real-life example, provided by a crisis pregnancy centre director:

> Recently a young woman came for a pregnancy test appointment. It wasn't only the test she wanted. She wanted someone to talk to. In fact, she repeated the test at home several times before coming to see us. She never thought she would get pregnant. She was hoping that the home tests were wrong, and the two telling test lines wouldn't show up again. She wanted to talk with someone confidentially to unravel the conflicting voices in her head that kept her tossing and

turning at night. She *couldn't* be pregnant and she wanted to know what she needed to do to get her life back to normal. Abortion seemed to be her only way out.

She told me about her situation. She was completing her second year of university with plans to become a professional in her field after three more years of study. Her boyfriend also had several years of school before he was to graduate. They were thinking of getting married but only once they finished school, had jobs and had money for a house. Both were living at home with their parents. She told me she was a Christian who regularly attended church, and had put her trust in the Lord Jesus Christ. I know and hold high regard for the church she attended.

I asked her what she believed about abortion. She believed abortion is wrong. In high school, she had participated in a pro-life club that held up curbside signs calling for an end to abortion. Even though she believed abortion was wrong, given her situation she believed she couldn't have a baby – that God wouldn't *want* her to have a child now. Fears of bringing shame on her family and on her church were the key factors influencing her to think that her abortion was necessary. She was aware she had crossed God's boundaries by being sexually active before marriage. She was willing to bear any personal pain that might come with an abortion – physical, emotional or spiritual, she just didn't want her church and family to suffer from her bad choices. **She convinced herself that abortion, in her case, was a self-denying act.** Even with her Christian background, at that moment, she could not feel her feet sliding down a slippery slope. She did not see that trying to cover her sexual sin by having an abortion could bring even greater harm to herself, not to mention ending the life of the child who God entrusted to her care.

"How is your faith helping you during this difficult time?" She sobbed and reached for a tissue.

"My life is over. How can I keep going to school and ever hope to be successful in life? I can't even remember to make lunch without my mom's help, how could I take care of a baby? I'm too young. We're not ready to be married. What if my parents found out I was pregnant? They would kill me. And they have already paid my tuition. If I show up obviously pregnant at my church my parents will have to step down from their leadership positions. Everyone will talk about us. I can't pray to God anymore. I hate this. ***I'm sinful by being pregnant and I'm sinful if I abort, so what's the difference?*** I have other friends who had abortions and they got over it. It will probably be hard on me emotionally but I really have no choice. And adoption? I could never do that. If I am going to go through the pregnancy I am not going to give my baby away to people I don't know. A baby should be raised by her own mother and father. If I can't be a good mother, abortion is best so the child doesn't have to suffer a terrible life. I don't want to, but you see I really have no other choice."

Were her arguments logical? Were they based on the truth of Scripture? No. Temptation to sin never is. In Romans 7, Paul speaks about the struggle of the flesh directing us away from God's protective and life-giving boundaries. As Christians in our daily struggle against sin we don't often fall because we don't *know* what the right action is. **Rather, we sin when we see the wrong action as being easier and more attractive.**

This account powerfully illustrates the destructive effect of sin on worldview and behaviour. Remembering Jesus' words in Mark's gospel, when sinful hearts see the murder of the innocent as an option, they are also open to deceit, foolishness, and a host of other evils. When we engage in pro-life advocacy, we are confronting people's most cherished lies; people often know, intellectually, that the pro-abortion position is destructive and illogical, but their commitments come *before*, and go *beyond*, mere rationality.

IN THIS BOOK

This short book is intended to equip Christians with a foundation of theological and philosophical reasons why the work of advocating for the rights of the unborn is critical, especially in our current cultural landscape in the West. How do we understand and articulate the biblical basis for the pro-life position? How should we respond to the killing of unborn children?

In these pages, we seek to answer such questions by providing a biblical and historical understanding of the idolatry which gave rise to our present culture's obsession with death, as well as a comprehensive, biblically-grounded rationale for why and how we may speak up for life. Finally, in opposing abortion,

Christians must also account for the experience of the vulnerable souls who are considering it, that we might be equipped to minister to them with compassionate understanding.

Precious Thoughts and Precious Life in a Culture of Death

While the worldview that promotes abortion is an ancient one, the flashpoint of the modern Western abortion movement is the Sexual Revolution of the 1960s. This ideological revolution set out to change *culture*, rather than politics, and regarded the Christian sexual ethics that had helped to shape Western society as "retrogressive and stifling and the enemy of The Good Life. Its goal was to treat sex as individual recreation, an end in itself.... Therefore, almost every form of adult consensual sex was normalized."[2] The *'pro-choice'* position, brought into the mainstream of culture by the Sexual Revolution, has had terrible, dehumanizing effects on women, children and fathers. It has led the Western world to regard women *essentially* as sex objects rather than as *persons*, whose sexual being is fulfilled in a monogamous, complementary relationship to their gender-opposite, in a covenant relationship of duties and responsibilities, which include those towards the unborn child.[3]

As a result of the Sexual Revolution and the changing social attitude to sexuality and family, our age is facing a fertility crisis because we are producing fewer and fewer children – an ideal promoted on every side, since children are increasingly seen as a drag on individual mobility, freedom and independence. Abortion has greatly contributed to these declining birth rates. As an aspect of the deep hostility amongst cultural elites toward the Christian view of the family, a culture of death is growing up around us. Most politicians still steadfastly refuse to address the issue of abortion in Canada, while the courts continue to imprison people engaging in peaceful Christian witness to protect life near the many abortion clinics.

Meanwhile, leading medical intellectuals writing in the *Journal of Medical Ethics* are calling for the legitimization of "after-birth abortion" (i.e. infanticide), for the same reasons someone would have an abortion now, declaring that the newborn infant is only a 'potential person,' without a moral right to life.[4] The British Medical Association has advised doctors that there may be grounds for abortion solely on the basis of the sex of the foetus. A recent investigative journalistic operation found that sex-selective abortion (i.e. the abortion of baby girls) was prevalent, even though it remains against the law. Subsequent inspections of clinics in the U.K found that the pre-signing of abortion forms by doctors, without any contact with the woman seeking to acquire an abortion, as well as the photocopying of doctors' signatures to pre-approve abortions, was widespread.[5]

This bizarre Western death-wish is propagated in one cultural message after another by media, film and educational materials, where we are perpetually told that humans are infesting the planet, destroying Mother Nature and using up her resources, so that ideas such as zero population growth, zero economic growth and carbon footprint reduction through any and all means, including abortion, have become political orthodoxy for many. Alongside this, our children in state schools are taught that sex is primarily for the purpose of recreation with anyone, not procreation; the killing of unborn babies is a mother's right; euthanizing the very sick and the elderly is compassionate; and governmental social engineering, not God, governs our lives.

PRECIOUS THOUGHTS

Into this contemporary chaos speaks the great I AM in Psalm 139 through David's marvellous prayer:

> O Lord, you have searched me and known me!
> You know when I sit down and when I rise up;
> you discern my thoughts from afar.
> You search out my path and my lying down
> and are acquainted with all my ways.
> Even before a word is on my tongue,
> behold, O Lord, you know it altogether.
> You hem me in, behind and before,
> and lay your hand upon me.
> Such knowledge is too wonderful for me;
> it is high; I cannot attain it.
>
> Where shall I go from your Spirit?
> Or where shall I flee from your presence?
>
> If I ascend to heaven, you are there!

If I make my bed in Sheol, you are there!
If I take the wings of the morning
 and dwell in the uttermost parts of the sea,
even there your hand shall lead me,
 and your right hand shall hold me.
If I say, "Surely the darkness shall cover me,
 and the light about me be night,"
even the darkness is not dark to you;
 the night is bright as the day,
 for darkness is as light with you.

For you formed my inward parts;
 you knitted me together in my mother's womb.
I praise you, for I am fearfully and wonderfully made.
Wonderful are your works;
 my soul knows it very well.
My frame was not hidden from you,
when I was being made in secret,
 intricately woven in the depths of the earth.
Your eyes saw my unformed substance;
in your book were written, every one of them,
 the days that were formed for me,
 when as yet there was none of them.

How precious to me are your thoughts, O God!
 How vast is the sum of them!
If I would count them, they are more than the sand.
 I awake, and I am still with you.

> Oh that you would slay the wicked, O God!
> O men of blood, depart from me!
> They speak against you with malicious intent;
> your enemies take your name in vain.
> Do I not hate those who hate you, O LORD?
> And do I not loathe those who rise up against you?
> I hate them with complete hatred;
> I count them my enemies.
>
> Search me, O God, and know my heart!
> Try me and know my thoughts!
> And see if there be any grievous way in me,
> and lead me in the way everlasting!

This well-known psalm is a personal petition to know and to be led by the infinite and ineffable God, though surrounded by the wickedness of ungodly men. The psalm celebrates God's intimate omniscience, His omnipotence, His omni-competence in all human affairs (otherwise known as providence), and His mercy and wonderful judgments. We have here presented to us the triune God who knows all men, their aims, purposes and desires, a God from whom nothing is hidden, and yet who enters into covenant relationship with His people using His personal name, I AM. We see that God tests and searches us as creator and king. And in particular, we are confronted with His absolute sovereignty, providence and predestination from womb to tomb.

THE INTIMATE PROVIDENCE OF GOD

The first verse of Psalm 139 literally reads, *"I AM, you*

searched me and you know me." This is worth reflecting on. The covenant God searches us, and He knows us better than we know ourselves. We see in verses 2-4 the comprehensive extent and exhaustive character of that knowledge. This kind of intimate, all-encompassing knowledge is beyond our ability to fully grasp; it is high and impregnable to our limited understanding, a wonder and mystery which humbles us, and calls us to bow before it (v. 6).

David reminds us that there is nowhere we can flee from the all-seeing omniscience of God – it hems us in (v. 5). There is no hiding place from the presence of God, neither in the heavens nor in the grave can we escape His intimate knowledge and sovereignty (v. 7-9). To the believer this is a great comfort, joy and delight, but to the enemies of God it is an intolerable terror and an insult to their self-professed autonomy *from* God. Our inability to escape God at any point or in any place is dramatically set forth in verse 8, which literally reads, *"If I spread out my bed in the grave, behold, you are there!"* John Calvin puts it well: people *"cannot move a hair's breadth without his knowledge."*[6]

This reality is powerful and important, but there is yet more to marvel at in this psalm. It is not simply that God *knows all things;* He is *involved.* As His covenant people He lays His hand upon us (v. 5). This is a hand of care and protection, as well as of judgment. For God to lay the hand upon someone here represents His full authority over all men. When I lay my hand upon my children, it is sometimes to protect or carry them, sometimes to restrain or discipline them, but it always exhibits my authority. This is why grabbing or restraining someone we have no right to control, against their will, can be construed as assault; it is an illegitimate exercise of authority.

Sometimes the biblical writers, like Job, call on God to *remove* His hand of discipline or judgment in the midst of His mysterious working, yet how grateful we ought to be, like the psalmist, for the hand of God even when it seems heavy upon us (cf. Job 6:9, 13:21). If it were not for the forceful hand of God whose authority and jurisdiction is total, Lot would have stayed in Sodom. Yet, by grace, when he lingered, the angels grabbed him by the hand and led him out. If it were up to us, we would have cradled and nursed our sins and remained in rebellion against God with stony and defiant hearts, but He calls us out of darkness into His marvellous light, raising us from spiritual death to life. Sometimes, God's hand is also upon us as He cares for and comforts us. It is an immeasurable mercy to know the comforting hand of God in all things. His ever-present, all-knowing and all-powerful work is unrelenting in every area of life – this is the personal *presence* of the Holy Spirit. Sometimes even Christians want to run away from this all-conditioning God. But David declares *"even the darkness is not dark to you; the night is bright as the day, for darkness is as light with you"* (v. 12).

GOD'S STUDIO

Nowhere is this mysterious, all-conditioning providence more dramatically illustrated than in the marvel that is human conception and gestation. At the centre of this great prayer is one of the most beautiful and important declarations in the Psalms, emphatically revealing the sanctity of life (v. 13-16).

So remarkable are these things that David declares, *"How precious to me are your thoughts oh God, how vast is the sum of them."* God's total providence and sovereignty are not simply seen in His pervasive presence and knowledge of our activities; they are manifest in His personal creativity and ordination within our lives, from conception to our last breath. Here therefore, creation and predestination (that is, God's calling) are seen to be involved in each other.

The womb itself is God's *studio*, poetically described as "the depths of the earth," a place totally hidden (v. 15). From conception through gestation, "you knitted me together in my mother's womb. I praise you for I am fearfully and wonderfully made. The psalm thus shows that we all were personally predestined in God's righteous will and called into being for the purposes of God; all of this manifests the grace and mercy of God.

In verse 16 we have another critical statement in relation to our subject of the sanctity of human life. The Hebrew text literally reads, *"My embryo (golmi) your eyes saw."* This phrase means an incomplete vessel; the life is young and unfinished. The rest of the verse then goes on to beautifully relate the active creation of the human embryo, in terms of God's predestination of the totality of life. The sovereign Lord has ordained our days and our steps: "in your book were written every one of them, the days formed for me, when as yet there was none of them" (v. 16). As if to reinforce this marvellous truth, the word "formed" carries the sense of the forming of a plan prior to its enactment. God is not just counting the days in His secret work, He is *forming* the future before our hearts begin to beat, giving meaning to every moment. Every person is thus fashioned in terms of God's holy purposes. Both the Old and New Testaments provide specific examples of this wonder. Consider Jeremiah 1:5: "Before I formed you in the womb I knew you, and before you were born I consecrated you;" and St. Paul in Galatians 1:15-16: "he who had set me apart before I was born, and who called me by His grace, was pleased to reveal His son to me."

GOD'S JUDGMENT ON THE WICKED

Following powerful statements about the all-conditioning providence and loving care of God from conception to the grave, we read King David calling on God to *judge* the wicked. David hands his life over to God as one formed for the purpose of doing battle against wickedness. These wicked men of blood come under the censure of God and David for their lawlessness. These lawless deeds include murder (v. 19), a violation of the Sixth Commandment, and blasphemy (v. 20), a violation of the Third Commandment. Verse 20 makes clear that there is premeditation, planning and forethought involved in their scheming against God. These murderers use the name of God as though He were on their side. Apostate churchmen are involved in blasphemy whenever they endorse or support what God condemns.

In verses often passed over in a consideration of this psalm, David declares *his* hatred of those who, in their murderous lawlessness, hate *God* (v. 21). This reflects God's own hatred of the wicked as seen in Psalm 5:4-6: "For you are not a God who delights in wickedness; evil may not dwell with you. The boastful shall not stand before your eyes; you hate all evildoers. You destroy those who speak lies; the Lord abhors the bloodthirsty and deceitful man." Grammatically, the term *hate* here means the strongest possible aversion to lawless works and the people who delight in them. David thus declares that he loathes those who in this way oppose, plan against, and rise up against God. Calvin noted of this psalm, *"Our attachment to godliness must be inwardly defective if it does not generate an abhorrence of sin."*[7]

We should not read in to this text a malevolent, vindictive, self-centred motive, or a merely emotional understanding of David's divinely-inspired words. He is pointing out that there is a real, spiritual battle between truth and falsehood, God and Satan, light and darkness, in which life and death are very literally at stake – in this conflict there is no middle ground, no irenic third way. According to the Scriptures, love is the fulfilment of the law (Rom. 13:8-10); Jesus' commandment to love our enemies must not be read as an impossible task of stirring up warm emotional connections to those people, but to obey God's law concerning them (Matt. 5:44). We do not steal from them or bear false witness against them, for example. Moreover, we obey the Lord's command to make known to them the gospel of Jesus Christ which calls them to repentance (Matt. 28:18-20). As law-abiding people, lawlessness must be a horror to us, or we cannot be a people of love. In this sense, then, to hate *the wicked* (not just lawlessness in the abstract) is an aspect of love to God, because love fears God and obeys His law.

Scripture requires that we maintain an abhorrence of evil and the strongest possible censure of those who hate and blaspheme God in their murderous ways. To approve of such people and their works is to participate in their evil. In Luke 14:26 Jesus said that if a person does not "hate his own father and mother and wife and children, brothers and sisters and yes, even his own life, cannot be my disciple." Obviously by this He did not mean we are to cultivate an *emotion* of hatred toward our family. Rather, Jesus taught us that if anything comes before God in our lives, even familial relationships, it is a form of idolatry. To fail to have the strongest possible aversion to the evil man in terms of God's law is to put sentimentality before what God requires, which is likewise a form of idolatry.

DESPOILING THE MASTERPIECE – KILLING THE FUTURE

Given, then, that the womb is the master craftsman's studio for sculpting the future, it is only when we have considered this *mercy* of God (the womb), and the providential care of God in the creation of the human embryo, that we can begin to appreciate the evil of abortion. One of the tragic ironies of abortion is that it constitutes murder *in the life of the family*, so that the cradle of life is turned into a place of death. Considering the Bible's clear teaching, the wickedness of abortion should be obvious to Christians. Yet, according to some polls, religious school students are just as likely to have abortions as their secular counterparts. Allegedly, one in four evangelicals in

America are "conflicted" on the question of abortion. The silence on this issue in the church is too often deafening (unless it is a voice *for* abortion, as a recent survey of *United Church Observer* readers found), because to address the subject is seen as 'political,' and politics, we are often told, doesn't mix with biblical faith.[8] Nevertheless the true church has long seen, in terms of biblical standards, the destruction of the human embryo as murder. The grounds for this are seen clearly in the Sixth Commandment ("you shall not murder") and in Exodus 21:22-25:

> When men strive together and hit a pregnant woman, so that her children come out, but there is no harm, the one who hit her shall surely be fined, as the woman's husband shall impose on him, and he shall pay as the judges determine. But if there is harm, then you shall pay life for life, eye for eye, tooth for tooth, hand for hand, foot for foot, burn for burn, wound for wound, stripe for stripe.

This is a case law that sets out, by a minimal case, certain applications and implications. Firstly, the case here is of an *accidental* abortion. If the penalty for causing an abortion, not by pre-meditated violence but by criminal negligence, is so severe, it is obvious that abortion deliberately induced is strongly forbidden. We see from the text that abortion carried with it the maximum sentence of death, and is therefore considered murder in God's law. Even if mother and child are not injured in the incident, the negligent man must be fined. In other words, God's law sets around a pregnant woman and her embryo a hedge of protection, second to none. In

Scripture even a mother bird with eggs or young is protected by the law, to prevent the exploitation of God's creation (Deut. 22:6); if birds are to be protected, how much more expectant mothers with their unborn child?

The challenge we face today in applying God's law to the matter of abortion is not new. The early church had to confront the widespread reality of abortion in the Greco-Roman world. The Greek philosophers were often advocates of both abortion and infanticide whenever they were perceived to be in the interests of the pagan state. Plato's *Republic* argues that the state is the ultimate order and functional god, and can order abortion, infanticide and incest as it sees fit.[9] Aristotle's ideal society required abortions when state-permitted births were exceeded.[10] Furthermore, in Roman law, abortion and infanticide were not essentially distinguished. Infants did not actually have legal status until the head of the family, the "*pater familias*," accepted the child into the family. Until that acceptance, an infant could be destroyed.[11]

By contrast, the early church quickly condemned abortion. Tertullian wrote: *"to hinder a birth is merely a speedier man-killing; nor does it matter whether you take away a life that is born, or destroy one that is coming to birth. That is, a man that is going to be one; you have the fruit already in its seed."*[12] The early Apostolic Constitutions likewise call for vengeance upon those who destroy the unborn child. So serious was this to the church that, because the Roman Empire did not see abortion as a crime in the way the Bible does, many church communities pronounced their own ecclesiastical sentence of 'penance for life,' to indicate the capital nature of the offence. The Council of Ancyra in ad 314 noted this earlier practice and limited the restitution/penance to ten years.13 Among the pagans, by contrast, Tacitus, the Roman historian and senator, found it repugnant that the Jews *would not* kill babies.

In many countries today, abortion and state control of births are not only legal, but seen as a basic right. As biblical faith has declined in the West, abortions have correspondingly increased. In Canada today, abortion is sponsored by the Ministry of Health, and permissible all the way up to full-term.[14] American research shows that the reasons most often cited for an abortion are people claiming they are "not ready for the responsibility," or "inadequate finances." 1% concern rape.[15] Other common motivations for having an abortion found in various studies include the preservation of beauty; the continued enjoyment of freedom and irresponsibility; a hatred of life; a hatred of men; and the alleged imperfection of a foetus. On the last point concerning the imperfection of a foetus, two American doctors, writing back in the 1960s, have rightly noted:

> No human being is perfect. Would the world, moreover, really be a better place after the destruction of the millions of defective individuals? Has the world gained or lost from the services of the epileptic Michelangelo, of the deaf Edison, of the hunchback Steinmetz, of the Roosevelts – both the asthmatic Theodore and the polio paralyzed Franklin? It must be recognized that liberalized abortion laws would logically be

followed by pressures for legalized euthanasia. The attack on life is essentially the same.[16]

This attack on life in general began with the abolition of laws against abortion, and the fight is escalating. Recently in the UK's *Daily Mail Online*, an article was published on the National Health Service (the UK's socialized medicine system), in the case of a doctor who has blown the whistle on the NHS allegedly euthanizing 130,000 elderly patients every year because "they are difficult to manage or to free up beds."[17]

These overt attacks on life are a modern form of eugenics – the attempt to control a supposed evolutionary process by controlling who reproduces and who is born. Hitler's sterilization laws and eugenics programs were modelled in the United States by the work and legislative preparation of American evolutionary biologist Dr. Harry Laughlin. The founder of the modern pro-abortion, birth control movement, (and Planned Parenthood) was the racist eugenicist, Margaret Sanger (1879-1966). A white supremacist, she even addressed a meeting of the *Ku Klux Klan*. She argued that *"the brains of Australian Aborigines were only one step more evolved than chimpanzees and just under blacks, Jews and Italians."*[18] Her early clinics were initially strategically located to control the births of Slavs, Latins, and Jews. She later targeted African American communities.[19] Planned Parenthood itself reported that of the 132,314 abortions it performed in 1991 in the USA, 42.7% were on African Americans and other minorities, even though they make up only 19.7% of the population.[20]

CHOOSE LIFE

Great spiritual evil is at work in the destruction of the life of the most helpless and innocent of all human beings. There is something profoundly malevolent in this wanton killing, a love of death that is basic to sinful man's spiritual condition. This orientation toward death, the Bible tells us, marks men and cultures that are in rebellion against God – that is, by their hostility to God they become suicidal in their inclinations (Prov. 8:36). Scripture tells us there is an inseparable link between sin and death. Spiritual separation from the source of life in Jesus Christ means a growing tendency toward death, because Christ alone is the resurrection and the life and the light that leads to life. Christ's atonement and lordship in our lives separates us from the power of sin and death, consecrating us to life and righteousness, for in Christ the power of death is broken (1 Cor. 15). In the pagan Greco-Roman world, into which this gospel was first declared, the great entertainment was death, paraded as games. Whether gladiators were fighting to the death or Christians were being tossed to lions, death was a spectator sport. As the gladiators entered the arena they cried, "Hail Caesar. We who are about to die salute you." The Christian faith eventually brought an end to the blood-letting and pagan sacrifices of the arena.

Not unlike the ancient Roman world, or the ideals of the Greek philosophers, morality today is being redefined in terms of whatever a statist elite says it is; life has value and is worth living when the state says so. The state has again made itself the ultimate order, and so abortion is consequently seen as simply a matter of politics, not God's law. The promotion of abortion is then, at root, a return to paganism and to a fundamental denial of the truth of Psalm 139. The psalmist asserts the total authority of the plans and purposes of God; in a retrogressive contrast to this in our day, the control of life by human agencies is the alternate plan of predestination *of man, by man.*

If we deny predestinating power to God in our thinking, we simply transfer that power to man and to the state (which is just man on a larger scale). Whenever belief in God's predestination declines, belief in the planning or predestination by the state over life and death rapidly takes its place. Abortion is thus an attempt to play God, to control, to grant, and to take life on man's own terms. It is ironic that modern humanism is against capital punishment for murderers (evildoers) where God requires it, but will exercise capital punishment against innocent unborn children whom God's law protects. If man can play God and write his own law, questions of life and death become open questions to be decided by the 'democratic will,' embodied by state planners and legislatures. Under God, the ministry of the doctor is meant to be a ministry of life and healing; under humanistic man-gods, doctors are increasingly being asked to become murderers. All this is done behind the blasphemous claim that humanism reverences and affirms life. But human worth, dignity and life are no longer affirmed or protected on the grounds that all human beings bear God's image; rather, the weak are murdered by the strong in the name of another human's right to choose. The psalmist makes clear that judgment looms over such an age dominated by 'men of blood' (v. 19), where God's name is hated and blasphemed.

ABSTRACTING EVIL

The reason we tend to find passages of Scripture like this difficult in our day is because many believers have unwittingly adopted the Aristotelian and humanistic notion of the division between intention and action, thereby depersonalizing sin by abstracting a man's *actions* from his true moral *nature*. Because life and history undeniably manifest real evil, it is only by resorting to pagan dualistic assumptions between intent (spirit) and act (matter), that humanistic thinking can retain the notion of a natural goodness or moral neutrality within man, over against the biblical doctrine of a fallen and sinful nature in all human beings, revealed by their deeds. This means that, as we see in Gnosticism, the spirit or mind can remain pure, while the material environment is thought to be impure, by nature inferior because of its dependence on the physical world. This being the case, many pagans thought that what you do in the body does not define your true moral character. People may say of a criminal, "yes, he is a murderer (or rapist, or pornographer or paedophile), but in his heart he's a good boy with good intentions." This sharp and artificial division of moral character from action seeks to preserve an anti-biblical view of man. It results in a denial of real responsibility whereby intent (or character) and act are divorced, rather than being seen as involved in each other. Works of evil can then be seen not as an expression of man's sinful and lawless heart, but as a form of strange social sickness produced by the person's environment, upbringing or lack of education.

Scripture makes clear, however, that sin does not have abstract, objective existence; rather sin is lawlessness and therefore is a moral quality *of a man (1 John 3:4)*. Sin is something *we think and do*. Murder and adultery are not things that have an existence apart from man. Crimes do not happen without a criminal – there is no sin without a sinner. Sin is not an idea, but an expression of a sinful and immoral nature. Murder is evil and so murderers are evil, since men do not murder out of the goodness of their hearts. Jesus made clear that a good tree does not bring forth bad fruit and *vice versa* (Matt. 7:18). Sin can and does manifest itself in thoughts, words and deeds, in historical events and their results, but it does not thereby gain independent metaphysical being – this would require the view that evil has a metaphysical ultimacy alongside God. This is why it is not sin in the abstract (merely as a category or idea) that the psalmist says we are to hate; we are also to have an established moral aversion of the strongest kind to evil men.

The Cosmology of Killing: Moloch Worship Repackaged

Given the inescapable reality of evildoers masquerading as righteous, it should come as no surprise that Christian morality in our time is increasingly rejected, sneered at as judgmental, hypocritical, or even an expression of hatred. To be faithful and wise witnesses in such a context, we need to relearn to understand our faith and make our case as the early apologists did amongst the pagans – not simply pragmatically, but cosmologically. The One who ordered all reality, who called it into existence, hallowed the womb by His incarnation, and the implications which flow from this fact are profound.

Two things are clear in Scripture. First, there really are *only two religions* and all people, necessarily, participate in one or the other – the worship and service of the *creator* or of the *creation*. And second, as a consequence, we are in a cosmic spiritual conflict that manifests itself in the ideas and practices of every social order. Social and cultural norms and practices are not neutral, coincidental or peripheral to fundamental beliefs (cosmology); rather they manifest our deepest religious commitments.

The roots of this go much further back than Greece and Rome, of course. We see it even amongst the Hebrews as they copied the pagans around them. As Jeremiah 32:33-35 makes plain, the Hebrews were drawn into the cult of creature worship and offered their children to Moloch. *Melek* is the common Hebrew word for *king* and is related to Moloch and Milcom, the god of the Ammonites, as explained in 1 Kings 11:7. A culture that exchanges the truth about God for *the lie* (Rom. 1:21-27) that man can be as god, is a culture that worships and serves creation, not the creator, and in the personification of nature with various gods (of which man is part), he in fact worships himself and his own will and idea, usually in the form of the state, a king or emperor. Moloch worship was in reality state worship – it was man worship. The brass statue of the god was in a human form with outstretched hands, and had a bull's head. A fire was stoked to incredible heat in the statue's belly and parents were required to offer up their babies to this terrifying embrace without any sign of protest, and then watch the horror unfold.

God's Word warns against this practice, and makes it clear that this was an aspect of religious paganism and occultism, in Deuteronomy 18:10-11:

> There shall not be found among you anyone who makes his son or his daughter pass through the fire, or one who practices witchcraft, or a soothsayer, or one who interprets omens, or a sorcerer or one who conjures spells, or a medium, or a spiritist, or one who calls up the dead.

Would it come as a surprise to learn that each of these occult practices are widely and actively pursued by many today in our culture, concurrent with abortion on demand? The cosmology of killing is thus pagan and occultic to its core, and originates in the first temptation, that man could be as God, determining good and evil for himself – to be beyond good and evil. The contemporary justification of the killing of the unborn, then, on the sole basis that it sanctions 'choice' (the woman's right to choose), is the essence of Moloch worship. We might not place our children in the fire, but the meaning, and the result, are the same. We satisfy self-will and the will of the state (man enlarged) by offering up our children on the altar of our own godhood, worshiping and serving the creature.

Our society, in abandoning the life-giving reality of the incarnation of the living Word, has adopted a cosmology of killing, in which we reveal Choice to be our god. We deny the reality of any value higher than our choice, and recognize no end greater than our will – all of which relates us to nothing but the existential self and therefore reduces us to nothing. As with the worship of Moloch, it is the 'free and voluntary' aspect of our killing that is the all-important basis of action in our pagan culture. And as we play god, the sterile and clinical abortuaries, with the states' strict limit on public protest around the killing centers, provide the deafening silence that shields mothers and cowardly men from comprehending the consequences of their actions.

To illustrate the fundamental cosmology of the pro-life position, let's briefly consider a cosmological critique of two common arguments for abortion: abortion as a matter of health, and as a matter of rights. The two are related. By identifying abortion as a human right, and thus an absolute, one of the more pernicious aspects of the contemporary practice of abortion in the West has developed: abortion has been identified as a matter of women's *health* and personal well-being. In the United States, the publications of the National Organization for Women (NOW) repeatedly refer to abortion as "the most fundamental right of women," *ahead* of the right to vote and the right to free speech. The protection of abortion rights is its top priority.[21]

ABORTION AS A DEFENSE OF WOMEN'S HEALTH

The common appeal to abortion as fundamentally a matter of 'women's health' is strange, if not altogether perverse. It does not matter whether health is understood physically, mentally or spiritually. While pregnancy does affect a woman's *physical* health, it cannot reasonably be categorized as if it were a form of *illness*, to be cured by excision. The natural 'cure' for pregnancy is a forty-week period of gestation that concludes in the birth of a child. It is a means of propagating the human race, and more specifically, the woman's kind. It thus obeys the first command given in Scripture: "be fruitful and multiply" (Gen. 1:28; 9:1). Associating abortion with 'women's health' cannot possibly refer to her *physical health*.

If not physical health, the identification of abortion with

health must refer to some sense of mental or spiritual well-being then. The facts speak incontrovertibly against its contribution to women's *mental* health. Dr. Priscilla Coleman recently published an article in the *British Journal of Psychiatry* surveying decades of studies, concluding that,

> Women who had undergone an abortion experienced an 81% increased risk of mental health problems, and nearly 10% of the incidence of mental health problems was shown to be attributable to abortion. The strongest subgroup estimates of increased risk occurred when abortion was compared with term pregnancy and when the outcomes pertained to substance use and suicidal behaviour.[22]

This leaves us with 'spiritual health.' If that is what is meant, it can only be a euphemism for child-slaying as a means of women's salvation, something akin to Moloch worship.[23] It represents a direct antithesis to the biblical text which speaks of a woman's salvation through child-bearing (1 Tim. 2:15).[24] Since the entire purpose of health care is the *preservation* and *furtherance* of life, the medical establishment ought to be seeking to abolish abortion rather than making an industry out of it.[25] At present, it breaks the Sixth Commandment in the name of fulfilling it, by appealing to 'choice.'

ABORTION AS A DEFENSE OF WOMEN'S RIGHTS

The appeal to the act of abortion as a centerpiece of *'women's rights'* is similarly nonsensical. Abortion cannot possibly be considered intrinsic to human nature or human flourishing. On the contrary, it strikes at the most *basic* human right, the right to life.[26] Killing abrogates all subsequent notions of justice and human rights. This 'woman's right' is by its nature *opposed to* human rights. It is not even intrinsic to being a woman, for it only appears at the moment when a child has been deprived of *its life and rights*. And many women would refuse to do so precisely for that reason.

What sort of claim is it then? The true nature of the claim that *some* people make can be seen in the argument typically used to attack a pro-life position: denying abortion forces women to have 'unwanted children.' One of the slogans for the pro-choice movement is 'Every child a wanted child.' Making a mother's *desire* the measure of a child's *worth* renders it a *commodity*. The woman's right to choose appears after the unborn child has been *depersonalized* and reconfigured as an item of *property*. It bears an uncanny similarity to the view of the 'rights' of the father in pagan Rome to dispense with his property as he saw fit. In both instances, the personhood of the child is denied, and the 'right' is exercised in the taking of another's life. This is in clear contravention of the understandings of human rights established by Christians in the West, largely to the advantage of women and children.

But the comparison between the choice of the ancient Roman father and present-day mothers only goes so far, precisely because of the advent of Christendom. Whereas the ancient world possessed no such notion as 'human rights,' that notion is the backdrop for the contemporary practice of abortion. There are only two ways in which the 'right to choose' to abort a child can be considered a matter of women's rights:

> i) Women's rights can be asserted if human rights are altogether suspended; or
>
> ii) They can be asserted if they lie *outside* the established understanding of human rights.

Both, I submit, have effectively happened. To allow for life to be taken by virtue of an appeal to a *different* set of rights is to assert the absolute priority of the latter over human rights. We are currently experiencing the consequence of allowing the state to define life in countless areas as a result. There is no logical stopping point to this process of abrogating human rights. More to the point, abortion rights not even resulted in the empowerment of women. Women have attained this absolute exemption to dispose of their 'property,' yet only under the condition that they too be similarly depersonalized; one of the most significant results of abortion rights has been the exclusion of women, legally speaking, from the human race.[27] The language of defending a woman's choice has nothing to do with her rights as a *person*. Proponents of women's rights defend 'what she can do with her body,' which is *not the same* as her person. Human personhood is a predicate of divine personhood. Detaching a woman's body from her person has rendered it a natural commodity that she possesses. Hence under *Roe v. Wade*, the ground for the legal change was construed to be the right to 'privacy' against any societal claims of jurisdiction.[28]

EVANGELICAL APATHY TO THE RETURN OF MOLOCH WORSHIP

Despite the horror of abortion, its cost of millions of lives, and the anguish it inflicts on countless others, it is still common to read among some of the most respected evangelicals of our day that culture is a matter of secondary concern, if not a matter of indifference, to Christians. The Christian faith is said to be solely a matter of 'winning souls.' The more extreme of the views parrot the moral relativism of their secular contemporaries in agreeing that Christians should not seek to 'impose their values on others' by a public outworking of their faith, even though the Great Commission demands precisely a form of that – through discipling the nations, which always has moral, legal and political dimensions.[29] The earliest Christian confession was not that Jesus is Saviour. It was that *Jesus is Lord*. Christ cannot be king without a kingdom. Nowhere is the moral bankruptcy of the Christian retreat from culture more evident than in the refusal of many Christians to actively oppose the slaughter of the innocents of our day, or to seek to overturn what Popes John Paul II and Benedict XVI rightly called our present age's 'culture of death.' The complicity of Christians in the Sexual Revolution against its biblical understanding is doubtless one of the main reasons for this. Having salved their consciences that compromises can be made in the area of sexual morality, it is easier to lose sight of the gravity of moral stipulations regarding life itself.

Post-Christendom in fact most closely resembles the return to a civilization that is alien, indeed absolutely antithetical, to that of the Lord of life. The abortion of the unborn is the flip-side to the Sexual Revolution. It is, as Douglas Wilson puts it, "Moloch worship *redevivus*." Abortion is part of an ongoing redefinition of what it means to be human, which is also marked by the orientation of sex towards gender, i.e. to nothing but a figment of our imaginations. Wilson wryly notes of the change, "Mothers cultivate childlessness, wives are male, and husbands are female. Other than that, everything is the same as it was."[30]

In the Christian community, many would doubtless dispute the analogy between the practice of therapeutic abortion on demand and the return to a species of Moloch worship. They might observe that there is no sense of the *worship* of Moloch (or any other god) in the contemporary practice of abortion. There is no cult, no ritual prostitution, no religion. All this is true. But the justification for murdering one's offspring on the sole basis that it sanctions 'choice' is the essence of Moloch worship. The only difference is that it is ourselves, rather than a 'god,' being propitiated by an expression of our will. But both practices plainly share something. They are captive to an idol, and in both cases, they exemplify the truth of Scripture, which declares that "all those who hate me love death" (Prov. 8:36).

THE REVEALING REFERENCE TO ABORTION AS 'CHOICE'

The uncompromising devotion to the abortionist cause marks out those that support it as a sort of cult. But what sort might that be? G.K. Beale, in his book *We Become What We Worship: A Biblical Theology of Idolatry*, suggests, based on Isaiah 6, that whatever people revere, they resemble, either for ruin or for restoration.[31] In the case of Moloch worship, the civilizations that worshipped that fearsome idol were horrifically savage, and they gave their progeny over to death. It is entirely correct to say that there is nothing resembling brass idols in our midst. But there is more to it than that. What people revere is whatever they hold to be ultimate reality, whether it is the triune personal God of Scripture, or something else.

What is the ultimate reality, the true cosmology? Christians would say that it is the triune, personal God of Scripture, but that is not the dominant perspective of the day. The dominant perspective offers a cosmological explanation of a materialist nature. The prevailing cosmological view of our day, the explanation for the very existence of life and the universe, is called the 'big bang theory,' whereby everything spontaneously emerged from a hydrogen explosion. It further resulted in the enormous complexity and diversity, and the interrelatedness of everything that exists. Now if we were to describe the assumptions that had been made in this theory, we would be compelled to admit that it presumes that *something can spontaneously come from nothing*, and that *anything can basically become anything else*. It doesn't matter if we want to add the biological theory of evolution to it, because the idea is basically the same, which is why the theories happily co-exist.

THE WILL OF THE GOD; THE GOD OF THE WILL
Fundamentally, this theory provides an intellectual template

for the absolute freedom of the will to declare that anything can become anything else. The consequence of this in the sexual realm is what we might call 'pomosexuality' – post-modern sexuality. It's like magic. The mirage of 'gay marriage' is a cardinal illustration of worshipping 'choice.' The autonomy of the choice is revealed in declaring that something that hadn't previously existed now does; the 'worship' is clear in the demand that it be publicly celebrated and legally recognized. On the other hand, reducing the *institution* of marriage to a *verbal definition*, and then excluding the procreation of children from that definition, is a reduction of a something to a nothing. Passing legislation thereafter to include variations on the 'definition' to make it more inclusive (as with same-sex marriage) can make them 'official,' but no more real or socially effective. Without children, they cannot perpetuate themselves. We can similarly talk as if 'gender' exists in contradistinction to biological sex, and can manufacture new genders to identify new trains of thought, but they are no more than willful expressions, which officialdom can only will that the general populace will, because they will it to be so. And the legal and educational system will duly oblige, because the one thing that both have demonstrated in recent years they believe in common is the absolute freedom of the will.[32] Arbitrarily determining human life to begin at some point other than conception does *precisely the same, for it is an outworking of the same cosmology.*

In short, the ultimate reality of our day is a very comfortable and infinitely plastic form of nihilism, the reduction of everything, however well-established, to be a matter of simple redefinition, even if it thereby refers to *nothing but our will*. Our society worships death because it reveals its choice to be its own god.

David B. Hart explained our society's chief moral value as the absolute freedom of choice, with this analysis:

> ...a society that believes this must, at least implicitly, embrace and subtly advocate a very particular moral metaphysics: the unreality of any "value" higher than choice, or of any transcendent Good ordering desire towards a higher end. Desire is free to propose, seize, accept or reject, want or not want — *but not to obey*. Society must thus be secured against the intrusions of the Good, or of God, so that its citizens may determine their own lives by the choices they make from a universe of morally indifferent but variably desirable ends, unencumbered by any prior grammar of obligation or value.... Hence the liberties that permit one to...destroy one's unborn child are all equally intrinsically "good" because all are expressions of an inalienable freedom of choice. But, of course, if the will determines itself only in and through such choices, free from any prevenient natural order, then it too is in itself nothing.[33]

It is in the very terms of the woman's 'right to choose' that we find the appeal to a God-concept.

HOSTILE WITNESSES IN THE CULTURE WARS

This has thus far been a pro-life portrait of the issue. Let us also consider the cultural analysis of someone who would support the pro-choice position. Michael Valpy, former Religious Affairs columnist for Toronto's *Globe & Mail* newspaper, is a respected analyst of the religious and ethical issues of our day. I will take his commentary on the legacy of Henry Morgentaler, Canada's most famous abortionist, to illustrate the broad cultural significance he sees in the pro-choice movement in Canada. It is necessary to begin with a bit of context.

On Dominion Day, July 1, 2008, Morgentaler was vested as a Member in the Order of Canada. The insignia pinned to his chest by former Governor General Michaelle Jean bore the Latin motto *desiderantes meliorem patriam*, "they desire a better country." It is from Hebrews 11:16, the motto of those who live by faith in Jesus Christ. For Morgentaler, receiving the award marked an extraordinary reversal of fortunes. When the Order was established by Queen Elizabeth II back in 1967, abortion was strictly illegal, and the Christian motto doubtless seemed appropriate to Canadians, if for some only as a gesture towards 'tradition.' Yet revolutionary change was coming. That same year, Pierre Trudeau was responsible as Justice Minister for introducing the landmark *Criminal Law Amendment Act,* an omnibus bill whose provisions included, among other things, the decriminalization of homosexual acts between consenting adults, movement towards the legalization of abortion, contraception, and lotteries, and the loosening of divorce laws. It became law of the land in 1968-69. Another country came with it.

Reflecting on Morgentaler's elevation five years afterwards, at the time of his death, Valpy opined that it had signified that "the door was firmly shut on institutional religion's engagement in the public life of the nation." It was part of the trajectory of what progressives call being on the wrong side of history:

> Between Pierre Trudeau's partial de-criminalization of abortion in 1969 (in the same piece of legislation that completely de-criminalized homosexuality and contraception) and the Supreme Court's ruling in 1988 declaring any criminalization of abortion to be unconstitutional, it became clear that absolutist teachings from the realm of the sacred would no longer be the determining factor in public morality and the nation's public life.[34]

The fundamental issue, though, is the religious implication of the honour: "What could have been a more definitive rejection of the church's teaching than the Governor General presenting Morgentaler with the state's highest honour?"[35] Valpy means more than the bare symbolism of the act. Honouring Morgentaler represented far more than honouring the man who brought about the legalization of abortion in opposition to the church. At issue in the abortion debate was the still larger issue of *who* defines what life is. It had been God. Who was it now?

For Valpy, the answer was clear. Morgentaler was the conduit for the *appropriation* of the church's and the family's historical mandate by the state. The state had now honoured a man who had conspicuously – even defiantly – honoured the state above God, indeed who had honoured it *as a god*. In 'rejecting the church's teaching' on life, it *celebrated the state's teaching on life*. It was therefore a moment of vast cultural and religious significance. Valpy clearly views history as an inevitable progression towards greater liberty and enlightenment, and in accordance with that, he identifies Morgentaler's elevation as a beacon of Canadian values to be the defining moment between two lords, two laws, and two worldviews in Canada.[36]

There is something undeniably correct in Valpy's summary. For him, Canada has effectively ceased to be a Christian country, because in its most *basic* understanding of human life, i.e. in its *definition* of life, it is no longer defined by Christian law. He understands, as all progressivists (and too few Christians) do, that by exercising the prerogative of defining life (as also in redefining marriage) the state has usurped the Lordship of Christ, His sovereign authority over life as its Creator *in every area*, which is symbolized by His definition of all human life and legal protection over it. And if God's predetermination of life and history has been rejected in Canada, as it once was in Israel before the exile, man's predetermination of life and history invariably ensues. It is not just a piece of legislation. It strikes at the very heart of all law. As in Europe, he exults, Christian culture has now been utterly *privatized*. Christian worship is still permissible, Christian culture, as expressed through the public outworking of the faith, is not.

Christians have been conditioned to believe that God's Word has nothing to say to "political" issues like abortion, and even though they are uncomfortable with the *status quo*, are quite willing to leave the issue on the backburner. Yet, allowing for the denial of God's predestination of human life to become Canadian law is necessarily to replace it with human predestination, and more specifically the government's total determination of all life. That is because what is at issue is the same as was involved in original sin. Original sin is not, as one so often hears, a matter of eating from fruit of the Tree of Knowledge and thus 'becoming as gods.' That is a Gnostic distortion of the text. In Genesis 3, Adam and Eve ate the forbidden fruit of the Tree of the Knowledge *of Good and Evil*. The detail of the text is crucial. 'Becoming as gods' thus meant that Adam and Eve took upon themselves the power of *moral determination*. They not only exercised dominion over the created order, but acted as if they could exercise dominion over the King of creation Himself. And the immediate moral consequence of their action was not only the sentence of death they received, but also that the first of their children, Cain, exercised his own moral determination by killing the second, Abel. They had achieved the quasi-divine power of moral determination. Yet it characteristically expressed itself in the choice to take human life. As the ancient Roman proverb would have it: *homo homini lupus*. 'Man is man's wolf.'

This is the current state of affairs. The sense of purpose that the Christian faith has inculcated into the Western understanding of history does not permit the progressivist to assign history a direction without a *director*. The Lordship of Jesus Christ has been replaced with the lordship of man, his sovereign authority over life and death, expressed in the State which, as Hegel once wrote, is the 'voice of God on earth.' Politics has returned to what it had been in the Western world before Christendom, a theological-political enterprise in which there is *no* separation of church and state precisely because the state once again exercises the prerogatives of the church, as it did before the advent of Christendom. This sounds surprising because every time the Christian faith is suppressed in the public square in our day, it is done in the *name* of the 'separation of church and state.'[37]

THE ABORTION OF FATHERHOOD – HER CHOICE, HER PROBLEM

One of preeminent social legacies of Christendom was the eradication of the idea (through legal and political means) that women were the property of their husbands. The Bible insisted on the covenant obligations of man to wife, and of father and mother to child, as the basis of the social good. The Enlightenment's principles of human autonomy and freedom (rather than personhood and the family) as the fundamental human categories seriously eroded that, and brought about a backlash in the twentieth century. The feminist movement largely encouraged women to understand themselves in similarly mistaken autonomous terms, understandably demanding equal rights in a variety of areas where men's obligations had been previously understood. But the right to choose to abort a child – and the perceived need for it – validate the patriarchal worldview which holds that women, encumbered as they are by their reproductive capacity, are inferior to men because pregnancy requires them to depend on men. The Sexual Revolution simply elevated this phenomenon to crisis-level numbers.

Having explored the connections of the Sexual Revolution with abortion, and observed it as a social symptom of extreme theological peril, we must also be mindful of the devastating effects of abortion on the entire family, but particularly on the women it allegedly liberates and heals. The irony of the situation could hardly be more acute. Throughout the Western world, abortion is held to be the most fundamental women's right. Canada sees itself as at the forefront of women's rights precisely *because* it provides unlimited, fully-funded access to abortion. But nowhere is it more obvious that supporting abortion is different than standing for women's rights than in the widespread practice of gendercide, the choice to abort the unborn simply because they are girls.[38] The hypocrisy of those who have called themselves defenders of women's rights has been well and truly exposed on this issue. They might sound the dog whistle of 'oppression' and 'imposing patriarchy,' and a Pavlovian pack of 'activists' might still bay and gnash their teeth.[39] But they now stand shoulder-to-shoulder with patriarchal societies. The point of principle is clearly about defending the 'pro-choice' position against *any limitation*. Unfettered access to death as a 'choice' is sacrosanct.

The Cosmology of Life and Compassion

Yet even if we disregard the practice of gendercide, we still find that, forty years on, abortion on demand has failed to liberate the overwhelming majority of women or promote their good. Instead, it has promoted the terms of the Sexual Revolution – uncommitted, anonymous sex without consequences – to the detriment of women. Giving pregnant women the *sole prerogative* of 'choice' is the final insult. For it has exempted men from any responsibility. *Covenant fidelity has been done away with.* The sperm donor and the drunken sailor have the same status, the same effective rights and obligations, as a dutiful husband who loves his wife and would seek to be a good father to his children. In short, women's power to 'choose' not only results in the slaughter of millions, it has made for the unprecedented cultural phenomenon of single mothers and fatherless children, a statistic that seems to rise by the year.

Not only has it given men a free pass, it has increased the stigma on women for carrying or aborting the child, precisely because 'her choice' means it's now *all* on her shoulders. Once women leave the silencing cordon of 'confidentiality' of Moloch's functionaries in the clinic, *they alone* will have to hear either the baby's cries on their own, or their peers' attacks on their 'irresponsibility.' It is not only men who will anathematize the pregnant woman. Pressure from families and friends, who know that they too will have to bear the consequences of the mother's allegedly *autonomous* decision, is often unbearable. The promotion of abortion as the pre-eminent human good declares nothing other than the depth of depravity in the world today. Those who hate the Lord of life love death.

In contrast to the pagan cosmology of death, the Christian cosmology is one of life and compassion. We are *pro-life* because God is life and the author of life. God's very being and nature is defined by *begetting*. The Incarnation reminds us that the Son, though born into the world at a certain point in history, is the *eternally begotten* of the Father. The wonder here is that the unity of the Trinity is a self-giving familial community of love. In the incarnation, where "veiled in flesh the godhead see," we discover this divine community. As creatures made in God's image, His familial nature is reflected in the human family, where out of the union of male and female, made in the image of God, *begetting* takes place and *generation* occurs and brings life. To abort begetting is thus contrary to the very nature of God, who has revealed himself in the familial categories of Father and Son. In the antithetical view, the cosmology of killing, there is no eternal begetting. Ultimate reality is not the triune God, a personal divine community, but only an impersonal, empty and lifeless unity of being or non-being. Hence death and annihilation is the goal of existence in pagan thought. Consequently, abortion becomes *logical* in an anti-Christian worldview. We can see from this that when opposing abortion, we are not moralizing, we are applying theological reality by describing the true God and the nature of the world He has made.

A final dimension to this must be added with regard to the nature of the gospel; an aspect that the incarnation of Christ so clearly sets forth. Christ is born into the world as a human being, as the last Adam and head of a new humanity. God's people would be 'born again' by the Spirit of God and become representatives of the new creation. The character of our salvation is therefore one of birth and generation. Human birth, in Scripture, becomes a type of the new birth – we must be born again. We are re-*generated* through the work of the Holy Spirit, by the imperishable *seed* of the word of God. By this we are given life and brought into the *family* of God (1 Pt. 1:23). Thus, to deny birth is to reject the new birth; to deny creation is to reject the new creation; and to deny the fruition of family is to reject the family of God. Abortion is a logical extension of the cosmology of death, but God's very being and nature, as well as the plan of salvation itself, militate, theologically, against abortion and contradict the practice.

In the cosmology of compassion, God is at work in all history by His providential and salvific work to bring about His life-giving purposes. Jesus said, "I have come that you might have life, and life in all its fullness" (John 10:10). John's prologue tells us, "In him was life and the life was the light of men."

This reminds us that the creation of life is God's work, not man's, and as such it is solely in His hands, so that life is always on His terms. God's terms are set out in His Word. The Sixth Commandment, by prohibiting murder, brings with it the positive duty to *promote life* and protect the innocent – in so doing we are fulfilling the law and working with God's purposes for creation. The cosmology of compassion calls on us to reveal the love and mercy of the triune God. This love is manifest not only in His eternal begetting and the incarnation of the Son of God, but also by the gift of life in every womb.

THE EVERLASTING WAY

We are all sinners, yet mercifully, our sin can be forgiven by and through the atoning death of Jesus Christ, when we come to Him in true repentance and faith; this includes the sin of abortion. Scripture is clear that because of the sinful nature, all have sinned and come short of God's righteous standard (Rom. 3:23). Some of God's greatest servants were guilty of murder and adultery, including King David, the author of Psalm 139, and yet they found grace and renewal. Thus, David does not condemn evil in this psalm out of a sense of self-righteous superiority. In verses 23-24 he prays, *"search me oh God."* This is to be our starting point as believers. Search me first, Lord, not others. We must ask God to try us and know our thoughts in His intimate omniscience. And, like David, in such a case we should be quickly aware that our own integrity, such as it is, is not enough, we can only stand in His righteousness. We must all be tried and searched by God and we all have need of Him to lay His hand of covenant faithfulness upon us to guard, guide, discipline, and preserve us. This is why David prays in verse 24, "see if there is any grievous (wicked/offensive/lawless), way in me," and then, "lead me in the everlasting way." What is that way? It is that way in which we pray God's right hand to hold us fast. It is the way of Christ, the way of obedience, the way of righteousness and justice, the way of the kingdom of God. It is the only way in which we can walk by the power of the Holy Spirit – it is the path that leads to life!

ENDNOTES

[1] Camille Paglia, "Fresh Blood for the Vampire," *Salon*, last modified September 10, 2008, http://www.salon.com/2008/09/10/palin_10/.

[2] P. Andrew Sandlin, *The Christian Sexual Worldview: God's order in an age of sexual chaos,* (Coulterville, CA: Center for Cultural Leadership, 2015), 20.

[3] It is telling that the Playboy Foundation was from the very beginning an advocate of abortion rights. Cf. Carrie Pitzulo, "The Battle in Every Man's Bed: Playboy and the Fiery Feminists," *Journal of the History of Sexuality* 17, no. 2 (2008): 259-289, 10.1353/sex.0.0004

[4] Stephen Adams, "Killing Babies no different from abortion, experts say." *Daily Telegraph*, www.telegraph.co.uk/health/healthnews/9113394/Killing-babies-no-different-from-abortion, accessed April 29, 2013.

[5] Holly Watt and Claire Newell, "Law does not prohibit sex-selection abortions, DPP warns." Daily Telegraph, www.telegraph.co.uk/health/healthnews/10360386/Law-does-not-prohibit-sex-selection, accessed October 29, 2013.

[6] John Calvin, *Commentary on Psalms,* vol. 5, trans. James Anderson, (Grand Rapids: Christian Classics Ethereal Library, 1849), 191, http://www.ccel.org/ccel/calvin/calcom12.pdf, accessed October 7, 2013.

[7] Calvin, *Commentary on the Psalms,* 191.

[8] Cf. Patrick Craine, "Poll: United Church members significantly more liberal than Canadian public on abortion, euthanasia," *Lifesite News,* accessed July 12, 2012, http://www.lifesitenews.com/news/poll-united-church-members-more-liberal-than-canadian-public-on-abortion-eu.

[9] Plato, *Republic,* trans. Allan Bloom (New York: Basic Books, 1968), Book VIII, 546a-547a.

[10] Michael J. Gorman, *Abortion & the early church: Christian, Jewish &*

Pagan Attitudes in the Greco-Roman World, (Downers Grove, IL: IVP, 1982), 20-25.

11 Allen Mason Ward, Fritz M. Heichelheim, and Cedric A. Yeo, *A History of the Roman People* (Englewood Cliffs, NJ: Prentice Hall, 1983), 35-38.

12 Tertullian, *Apologia* 9.6. http://www.ccel.org/ccel/schaff/anf03.iv.iii.ix.html, accessed October 7, 2013.

13 Council of Ancyra, Canon 21, in *Nicene and Post-Nicene Fathers,* Second Series, Vol. 14. Translated by Henry Percival. Edited by Philip Schaff and Henry Wace (Buffalo: Christian Literature Publishing Co., 1900.) Revised and edited for New Advent by Kevin Knight, http://www.newadvent.org/fathers/3802.htm.

14 In 2015, (the most recent statistic available) there were 100,104 registered abortions that our taxes paid for. "Statistics - Abortion in Canada," *Abortion Rights Coalition of Canada,* accessed April 5, 2017, http://www.arcc-cdac.ca/backrounders/statistics-abortion-in-canada.pdf.

15 "Abortion Statistics," *Orlando Women's Center,* http://www.womenscenter.com/abortion_stats.html, accessed November 5, 2013.

16 A.C. and Norbert J. Mietus, "Criminal Abortion: 'A Failure of Law' or a Challenge to Society?" *American Bar Association Journal,* October 1965. Vol 51, no. 10: 926.

17 Steve Doughty, "Top doctor's chilling claim: The NHS kills off 130,000 elderly patients every year," *Daily Mail Online,* accessed June 19, 2012, http://www.dailymail.co.uk/news/article-2161869/Top-doctors-chilling-claim-The-NHS-kills-130-000-elderly-patients-year.html.

18 Carl Wieland, *One Human Family: The Bible, Science, Race and Culture,* (Powder Springs, GA: Creation Book Publishers, 2011), 65.

19 H.A. Washington, *Medical Apartheid: The Dark History of Medical Experimentation on Black Americans from Colonial Times to the Present* (New York: Doubleday, 2006), 196.

[20] Wieland, *One Human Family*, 65.
[21] In a 1999 speech celebrating the 30th anniversary of the passage of Trudeau's omnibus bill C-150, Senator Lucie Pépin similarly argued that its abortion legislation provided a new freedom which "proved to be a stepping stone for many other freedoms and options that have altered women's place in [Canadian] society — self-esteem, education, jobs, a voice and empowerment." See Debates of the Senate, 2nd Session, 36th Parliament, Vol. 138 no. 7: http://www.parl.gc.ca/Content/Sen/Chamber/362/Debates/pdf/007db_1999-11-16-e.pdf.
[22] P.K. Coleman. "Abortion and Mental Health: Quantitative Synthesis and Analysis of Research Published 1995 — 2009." *The British Journal of Psychiatry,* 2011, 199: 180–186. http://bjp.rcpsych.org/content/199/3/180.full.pdf+html
[23] Theologically, healthcare is a priestly function with salvific connotations that are related to the nature of the God who is worshipped. Cf. Joe Boot, "Health, Salvation and the Kingdom of God," *Jubilee* (Spring 2012).
[24] I take this difficult text to refer to the fulfillment of the dominion mandate – faithful women shall, through their obedience to the first commandment given to mankind, to 'be fruitful and multiply', inherit God's blessings in this life in anticipation of its fullness in the **eschaton.**
[25] The heart of the pro-life position resides in its obedience to the Sixth Commandment, as Qs.135–136 of the *Westminster Larger Catechism* make clear.
[26] For example, the *U.S. Declaration of Independence*, which asserts that "all men are endowed with certain inalienable rights," and that "among these are *life,* liberty, and the pursuit of happiness;" Article 3 of the 1948 *U.N. Declaration of Human Rights*, "Everyone has the right to *life,* liberty and security of person;" and the *Canadian Charter of Rights*

and Freedoms, Sect. 7: "Everyone has the right to *life*, liberty and security of the person and the right not to be deprived thereof except in accordance with the principles of fundamental justice."

[27] The right to life mentioned in Section 7 of the *Canadian Charter* stands, in clear reference to the U.N. declaration, as the basic right to be alive. The courts have lacked consistency in defending this. They ruled in the 1989 case of *Borowski v. Canada (Attorney General)* that the unborn were not subject to this protection due to mootness, i.e. *because they declined to decide*. On the other hand, in the 1993 case of *Rodriguez v. British Columbia (Attorney General)*, they rejected assisted suicide because the right to bodily control could not trump the right to life. It was a common societal belief that "human life is sacred or inviolable," and therefore security of the person itself could not include a right to suicide; suicide would destroy life and thus be inherently harmful. Instructive, and worrying, was the appeal to the shifting sands of 'societal beliefs' rather than any reference to something inalienable.

[28] At root, there are two different systems of law. The law that defends persons stems from the common law tradition. The law that defends 'privacy' stems from the Romantic idea of 'natural rights'.

[29] Perhaps the most alarming manner in which the church has followed the world is in allowing its teaching to follow the progressive methodology so ably described by C.S. Lewis in *The Abolition of Man*. Teaching has to some degree been allowed to separate from moral conduct and example.

[30] D. Wilson. "Delenda Est." *Blog and Mablog*, September 26, 2013. http://dougwils.com/s7-engaging-the-culture/delenda-est.html

[31] Downers Grove, IL: IVP Academic, 2008.

[32] In early October, the 60,000-strong *Thomson Reuters* media empire, in an effort to determine its diversity success, has asked its staff of

reporters, researchers, marketers and others to pick their sex from nine choices, including 'genderqueer,' a category for identities other than man or woman, and 'not sure'. http://washingtonexaminer.com/article/2536814

[33] D.B. Hart. "Christ and Nothing." *First Things*, October 2003. http://www.firstthings.com/article/2007/12/christ-and-nothing-28

[34] M. Valpy. "Morgentaler's Other Legacy — The Wall between Church and State. Posted June 3, 2012. http://www.cbc.ca/news/canada/story/2013/05/30/f-vp-valpy-morgentaler-religion.html

[35] Strictly speaking, the Order of Canada is not Canada's highest honour (the highest, the Order of Merit, is awarded at the monarch's prerogative), and Morgentaler was awarded the lowest of the three grades in the Order.

[36] Historians refer to this perspective as the Whig interpretation of history.

[37] The comment of his successor as Liberal leader, Michael Ignatieff, is telling: "A sovereign is a state with a monopoly on the means of force. *It is the object of ultimate allegiance and the source of law*." Ignatieff, like all Hegelians, divinizes the state. http://www.theglobeandmail.com/news/world/michael-ignatieff-911-and-the-age-of-sovereign-failure/article594094/

[38] Cf. Mara Hvistendahl's *Unnatural Selection: Choosing Boys over Girls and the Consequences of a World Full of Men* (USA: Public Affairs, 2011) speaks of a shortfall of 160 million girls in Asia, and the ills of the practice of 'choosing' one's offspring in general, an effect that has also been noted throughout the Western world. Last modified June 15, 2011: http://www.npr.org/2011/06/15/137106354/in-asia-the-perils-of-aborting-girls-and-keeping-boys

[39] In fact, the American Civil Liberties Union argued that a law that sought to make it a felony to knowingly provide a sex- or race-based

abortion was both sexist and racist. Cf. http://www.huffingtonpost.com/2013/05/29/arizona-abortion-ban-race-sex_n_3355493.html

www.ingramcontent.com/pod-product-compliance
Lightning Source LLC
Chambersburg PA
CBHW052136010526
44113CB00036B/2282